Brain Power

How to Nurture and Nourish

Your Brain for Top Performance

Ron Kness

Legal/Disclaimer Notices

Published by:

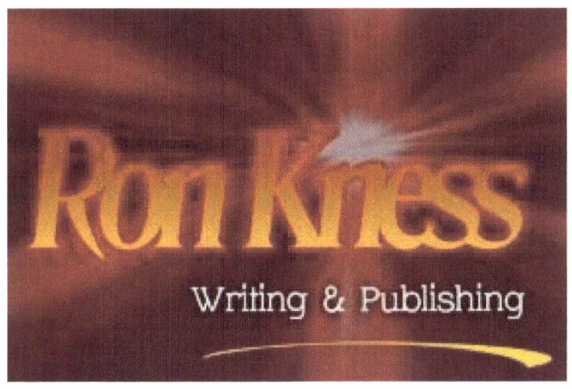

https://ronknesswriting.com

Ron Kness

San Tan Valley, AZ

United States of America

ISBN: 9781095328545

Brain Power Contents

Introduction

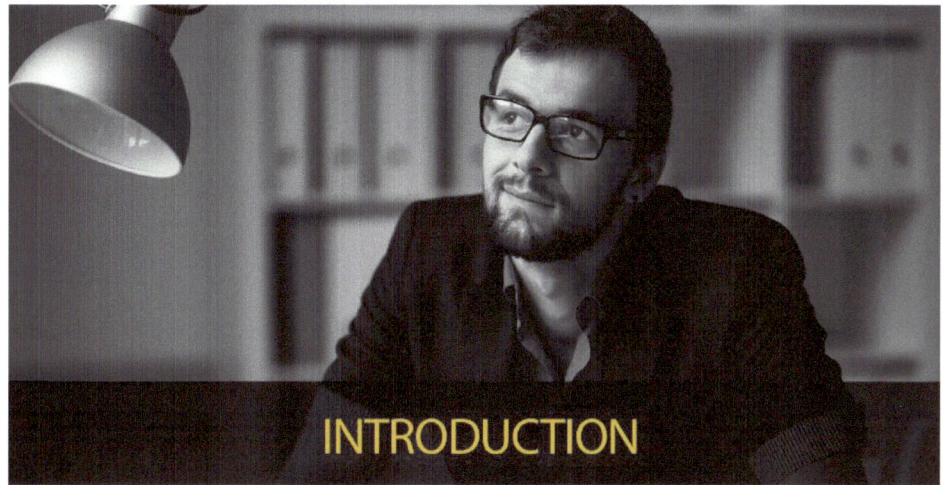

A lot of people are interested in health and fitness these days and to that end, they will spend a lot of time in the gym or out running in a bid to try and build more muscle and increase their physical fitness.

But while this is an admirable aim, it's maybe an example of us having the wrong priorities. Why? Because these days we don't use our bodies half as much as we use our brains. Our brains are what we use for the majority of careers these days, they are what we use to manage our relationships and they are what we use to handle money, navigate, learn and more.

So if you're going to spend time training your body, it only stands to reason that you should spend *at least* the same amount of time training your brain.

So why *aren't* more people already training their brains? Largely, this comes down to the fact that many people don't realize quite the extent to which their brains *can* be trained, or quite the extent to which their brain function can be improved through simply following the best health practices – through the right nutrition, lifestyle and more.

And more to the point, most people are completely unaware of just how *unhealthy* their current routine is for their brain. They have no idea that the things they're doing every single day are actually *damaging* their brains. And not only does this prevent those people from performing optimally every day but it could also lead to a higher chance of dementia or Alzheimer's.

Just think what you could accomplish if instead of degrading and abusing your brain, you instead focussed on nourishing it, training it and helping it to grow. You might just become limitless...

What You'll Learn in This Book

As mentioned, most people have at some time shown a basic interest in improving their physical fitness and strength. For this reason, most people have at least a *basic* idea of what fitness training entails and how to look after their body's health.

But seeing as brain health is a far less understood topic, this is an area that many people actually lack even basic knowledge of!

This book then will serve as a basic primer and introduction to your brain, as well as an advanced guide to how you can develop it and nurture it. We will cover everything from the basics of how the brain functions and good nutrition, all the way to much more advanced topics such as smart drugs and 'embodied cognition'.

You will learn:

- How your brain works
- The nature of intelligence
- How brain plasticity changes *everything* we once knew about the brain
- Why the right nutrition is crucial for optimum brain function
- The best lifestyle practices for increasing intelligence and improving performance
- How to increase focus and concentration
- How to train your body to train your mind
- How to use the right kind of brain training to enhance your cognition

- How nootropics work, who is taking them and whether you should take part
- Psychological tricks like CBT to help your brain work for you
- The power of meditation
- How to increase brain power by electrocuting it...
- Top things you need to STOP doing to avoid damaging your brain
- And MUCH more

By the end, you will have a far fuller understanding of your own brain and how to make the most of it. As a result, you can start to improve specific aspects of your brain, as well as its overall function. This will have *huge* impact on pretty much every area of your life as you become more effective in social settings, less tired, more sympathetic toward others (and better able to manipulate their emotions and thoughts), more attuned to your own strengths and weaknesses and more.

Once you learn to upgrade your own brainpower, you can trigger exponential improvements in every area of your life.

Are you ready for that change?

How Your Brain Works

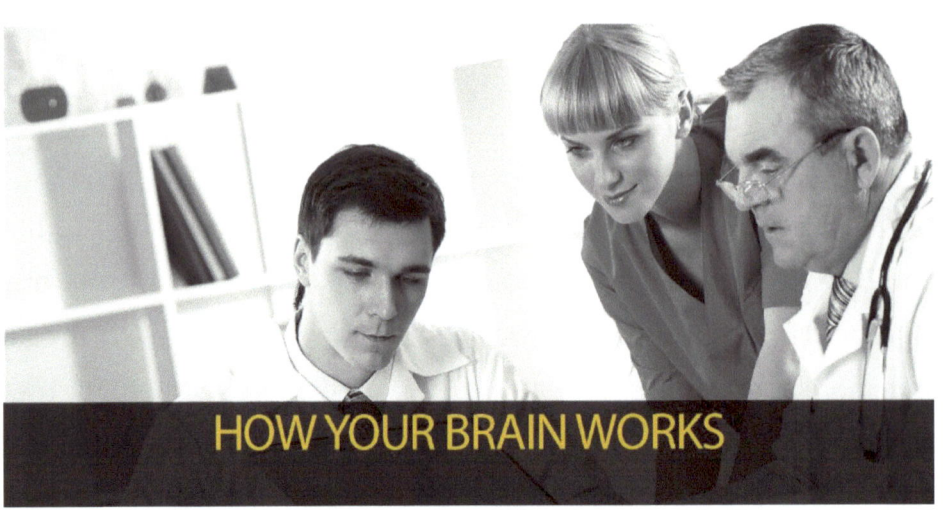

HOW YOUR BRAIN WORKS

The brain is by far the most powerful computer on the planet with billions upon billions of connections and a near limitless storage capacity. There are still countless things that we don't fully understand about our brains but nevertheless we *are* starting to understand more and more over time. And with each new discover comes new ways to get more from our grey matter and upgrade our performance.

The good news for you is that all this information is freely available now and you don't have to go through years of complex experiments and research to unlock all the secrets. In fact, this chapter will serve as a complete primer to bring you up-to-speed on your brain...

But a word of warning: this is complex stuff. If you *just* want to get to the good stuff and start learning how to get more from your brain, then you can skip this chapter. However, I highly recommend that you do *not*, seeing as it will give you a far better understanding of what's actually going on inside that skull of yours and thereby give you more autonomy when it comes to discovering new ways to tap into your cranium's near-limitless potential.

Neurons

The first thing to understand then, is that your brain is made up of billions of neurons. Neurons are 'brain cells' and in a sense, they operate just like any other cells in your body. They have a cell membrane (the wall surrounding the cell), they have a soma (the body of the cell) filled with cytoplasm (fluid), they have mitochondria to provide energy and they have a nucleus containing your DNA.

But brain cells also have a few 'extras'. Specifically, brain cells have axons and dendrites. The axons are the long 'tails' of your brain cells which protrude from the back. The dendrites meanwhile are a lot like routes or tendrils that stretch out across the brain coming off of the soma. The job of the dendrites is to find the axons of other cells, where they can then form a connection.

Neurons come in all shapes and sizes. While they are microscopic, they will sometimes have connections stretching all the way from one brain 'regions' to another to form connections. Brain cells don't actually touch but instead leave a small gap called the 'synaptic gap' and communication then occurs *across* the gap.

When a brain cell lights up or fires, this is called an 'action potential'. During this point, a small electrical current jumps from the synaptic 'knob' over to one or several connecting dendrites. This is how signals find their way around the brain.

Each time a neuron fires like this, it corresponds to some kind of subjective experience in the brain. For instance, one area of the brain – the occipital lobe – deals entirely with vision. When neurons in this region fire, it causes specs of light to appear like 'pixels' in the eyes of the viewer. Meanwhile, other neurons might make us remember a specific event, experience a smell, move a finger or fall asleep. Generally, neurons are arranged into groups which is what gives the brain distinct 'regions' for particular activity like this. At any time, you'll have a certain amount of activity in different regions of the brain – the entire brain is never lit up simultaneously. This will likely correspond with what you're thinking, what you're seeing and what you're feeling at any given time. And the connections mean that seeing one thing will often result in you remembering something else, or making the decision to do something.

Note that neurons only fire at one 'amount'. That is to say that there are no 'degrees' of firing – a cell is either firing or it is not. However, it might require input from numerous different surrounding neurons before it becomes excitable enough to light up itself.

Neurotransmitters and Hormones

But it is not just a current that jumps across the synaptic gap during communication between cells. At the end of each axon at the synaptic knob are tiny 'sacks' called 'neurovesicles'. These contain neurotransmitters, which include the likes of dopamine, serotonin and norepinephrine.

Basically, a neurotransmitter will change the excitability of your brain, the likelihood of memories forming, your attention or your mood.

For example, serotonin is the 'feel good' neurotransmitter. This means that it will normally be released when we see, think about or otherwise experience something that makes us happy. It's also released during exercise and when our body detects sugar!

Meanwhile, dopamine is a neurotransmitter that gets released when we think something is important. This then increases motivation, focus and the likelihood of a memory forming afterward.

Neurotransmitters in this sense tell us what we should be feeling about the experience of certain neurons firing. In some cases, a hormone can act like a neurotransmitter and vice versa. For instance, testosterone has an effect on our brain cells, as does cortisol. More often, neurotransmitters simply make a cell more or less likely to fire an action potential, which results in them being categorized as either 'excitatory' or 'inhibitory'.

In order for neurotransmitters to have an effect on us, they need to interact with 'receptors' located on the dendrites of cells. In other words, a neuron might release serotonin from its vesicles when it fires but this will only have any impact on those connected neurons that contain serotonin receptors.

Brain Plasticity

Once upon a time, scientists believed that the brain would be set in stone after a particular age. In other words, it was thought that once we reached adulthood, the brain would no longer continue to grow or change shape.

However, this has subsequently been found to be *way* off the mark. In reality, our brains continue to grow and change almost endlessly as we get older and this is how we are still able to formulate new memories and learn new subjects.

New brain cells can form in numerous regions of the brain for instance via a process called 'neurogenesis'. At the same time, new connections can also be formed and there is a simple rhyme to help you remember the rules here: 'neurons that fire together, wire together'.

In other words, if you *repeatedly* hear a particular sound while experiencing a particular smell, you will eventually get to the point where those two neurons form a connection. Over time, that connection will become stronger and stronger via a process called 'myelination'. Essentially, the axons and dendrites involved in the connection become better insulated, which strengthens the circuitry and makes it easier for one neurons to cause the other to fire.

This is how we can end up rote learning particular movements to the point where we no longer even need to think about them. One movement simply triggers the next movement automatically and almost without our conscious input.

Understanding brain plasticity – also known as neuroplasticity – is one of the most important secrets to improving your brain function. This is the mechanism through which all learning occurs and thereby, it can be tapped into to gain a huge number of new abilities!

What Our Brain Was Designed For Verses How We Are Using It

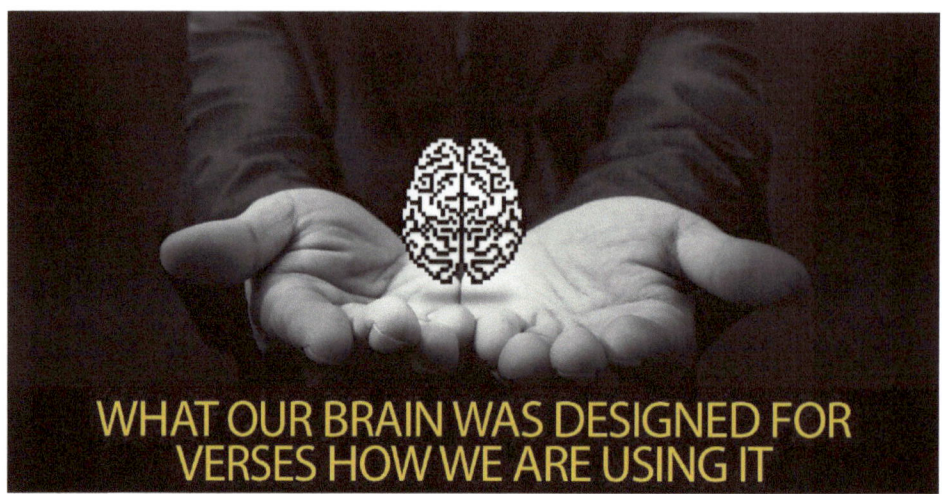

This basic primer has hopefully given you a good idea of how your brain works on a day-to-day basis and you're probably already seeing ways that you can improve its function: by increasing the number of desirable neurotransmitters for example, or by forming new connections by repeatedly performing two actions together that you want to become associated.

But what can also help a great degree is to understand what the brain was designed for and thereby *why* it is built the way it is.

And this all comes down to evolutionary psychology...

You Are an Adaptoid

The most important thing to understand about your brain is that it is built for survival. And how do you survive? By adapting to your environment. Every single aspect of your brain function is tied to this basic principle and that means that a lot of the way your brain works can be predicted in different circumstances.

At one point during the development of modern psychology, a field called 'behaviorism' reigned. What this school of thought basically told us, was that everything could be rote learned and that our entire subjective experience of the world was based on associations we formed through our interactions with the world.

The most famous example of this principle in action was the study referred to as 'Pavlolv's Dogs'. In this study, Ivan Pavolv rang a bell every single time he fed dogs. Over time, he found that the dogs would develop a response to the sound of the bell – they would begin salivating even when there was no food present. This demonstrated that they learned through association and that the simple repetition was enough to form that association.

Behaviorism says that everything we know is learned in this way. As babies we are largely 'blank slates' (though not entirely) and thus we learn how to interact with the world through association. For example, we learn that by reaching for things we will often be passed them. Thus we develop an understanding for the reaching gesture. When we touch fire, it causes a burning sensation, and the association that forms teaches us not to touch flames again. When we eat, it releases serotonin and we learn that we like eating. We come to associate the smell of cookies with Grandma's house and we learn language by seeing how people react to different words.

On a neural level, we now know that this is all to do with neural plasticity. Once again – what fires together, wires together. And when something is very important (like the fire), dopamine and other neurotransmitters are released to make that memory form even faster.

Our environment is always changing and thus this is the best way for the brain to survive. By adapting to different environments, our brains ensure that the behaviors we acquire are perfectly suited to the environment we're in. Ultimately, we learn to avoid danger and gravitate toward food, sex and shelter.

Why is this so important to understand? Because we're adapting to *any* situation we're put in. That means that you're still adapting right now to working in an office, being constantly stressed and looking at your phone a lot. The connections you're not using are atrophying, while many *unhealthy* behaviors continue to strengthen with time.

Enter: CBT and Embodied Cognition

But while behaviorism did a fine job of explaining psychology for a long time, it was eventually found to be overly simplistic and unable to explain the full gamut of human experiences. For instance, most of us would agree that we can learn things by *reading* for example. How does this fit into the behaviorist model?

And how can you become phobic of heights without ever having fallen from a height?

CBT (cognitive behavioral therapy) uses behaviorism as a starting point and then builds a cognitive element on top of that. This states that what we *think* also plays an important role – and that we can actually create new associations *by* thinking. In other words, if you think about falling, then this can create new neural connections as though you *were* falling – and that in turn can lead to the formation of a phobia, or to changes in personality.

Hold that concept in your mind for a moment while we take a look at another concept: this one is called 'embodied cognition'.

Embodied cognition is a more recent psychology theory that says *all* of our understanding of the world around us comes from our bodies. This fits with the evolutionary explanation that our brains evolved to help us survive in our environment based on our interactions.

The question that was posited to psychologists was this: when someone tells you some information, how do you understand that? You learned English growing up, yes, but what is it that allows you to understand *English*? Your brain doesn't innately understand English, so you must be 'translating' that language into something like a machine code in order to process it. For a while, psychologists made up the term 'mentalese' in order to explain this gap.

But later a more useful theory was put forward. Embodied cognition explained that we understand language by relating it *back* to our understanding of the world around us.

When you hear someone telling you a story about walking through a cold forest, you understand that by imagining *yourself* walking through a cold forest and this causes all those relevant neural connections to fire as you think of the implications of that, relevant memories *etc.*

And what's actually happening here, is that the areas of your brain are firing as though that story was really happening to you. If you put someone under an MRI scanner while you tell them about the time you went swimming, their brain areas will light up as though *they* were going swimming.

And this is how simply imagining something or picturing something can create associations in your brain. If you are high up and you keep *imagining* falling off that height, then your neurons will fire at the same time as though you *were* falling off that height. This is enough to cause those neurons to wire together and to create a strong connection – to the point where it's hard *not* to picture falling off of that height. This causes a flood of neurotransmitters related to the experience of falling and what do you know – you pass out in a sweaty heap!

CBT is a technique you can use to create more positive associations and connections in your brain and we'll look more at how this works later on in the book.

How to Train Your Brain for More Power

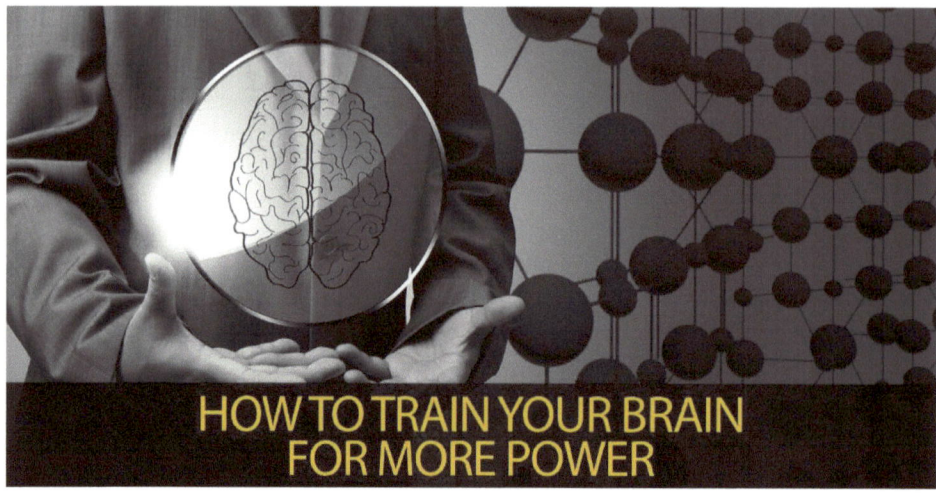

Understanding all of this, it's easy to see how brain training can work in theory – by helping you to create stronger connections throughout your brain and to create new connections entirely – thereby learning new skills and improving those you have.

And this is what has given rise to a lot of brain training programs and sites that teach you to do things like performing maths tests or memory challenges. The more you do this (in theory), the more you strengthen those skills and the better your memory, attention or mental arithmetic will become.

Which sounds like a seal of approval! So should you go ahead and start using that kind of brain training?

I argue no.

While something like Lumocity or Nintendo Brain Age might be useful for challenging you're recall or your special awareness, the reality is that they are far too *specific* to be all that useful in the real world.

When you train yourself to become better at spotting the number of cute penguins in a group (this is the kind of setup these fun brain training games often introduce), you become better at doing *precisely* that. You're strengthening neural connections *around* penguins. You're repeating that game over and over again and becoming better *at that game* – but this isn't going to do much for your ability to think of answers in an interview. It's not transferrable to 'real world' skills and for that reason, it's not going to be much use.

You know what *is* a good way to train yourself to become better at interviews though? Simple: expose yourself to more interviews! This will put you in the specific set of circumstances you need to enhance that skill and it will ensure you're using the precisely correct neural pathways.

But that's not to say that all brain training is a waste of time…

The Very Best Form of Brain Training

The very best form of brain training there is, is simply to challenge yourself to perform numerous different cognitive tasks and to continuously expose yourself to novel situations and challenges.

In other words, you need to consistently try new things, consistently test yourself and force your brain to keep on growing. The more you exercise your brain plasticity, the easier it will be and the more dopamine, norepinephrine, brain derived neurotrophic factor *etc.* you will produce.

It's only when you stop learning new things and stop challenging yourself that your brain becomes incredibly *un-plastic* and you begin to lose abilities.

Because brain plasticity *can* work both ways. A form of 'pruning' does occur when you go for a long time without using a specific neural pathway and that's why we are inclined to forget things over time. What's more, is that the brain will eventually stop producing neurotransmitters that enhance neuroplasticity. Brain derived neurotrophic factor (BDNF) and dopamine are directly related to myelination and neurogenesis (the creation of new brain cells) but if you never use them, they will occur less regularly.

A happy brain and a healthy brain is a brain that you are using in *lots* of unique ways.

Think about what an amazing learner you are as a baby. Why is that? Partly, this is due to the fact that *everything* around you is novel. The world is filled with things you don't understand and the brain is flooded with neurochemicals in order to start making sense of it all.

As you get older, more connections are created and you understand the world more. However, you will still continue learning lots of new things and experiencing lots of new things: as you go to school and college, as you move home, as you go through puberty, when you learn to drive, when you try out new hobbies...

But then you reach adulthood. You find a happy relationship, you fall into a job you like and your life finds a rhythm. You do that same job, day in and day out for the next 50 years. And the older you get, the fewer new experiences you expose yourself. You stick with the same friends, you stick at the same hobbies... and your brain stops growing.

And it's this that can eventually lead to danger as you become more likely to experience age-related cognitive decline or brain disorders like Alzheimer's or dementia. If nothing else, you become more forgetful, more set in your ways and less able to learn more skills.

And this is one reason that fluid intelligence (intelligence as opposed to knowledge), deteriorates as we get older.

But it doesn't have to be that way! Not if you understand how important it is to keep exposing yourself to new things and to keep learning.

Keep learning new languages. Learn new games. Meet new people. Explore new places.

Even just being in a novel environment will cause a flood of neurotransmitters associated with attention and awareness to fire. Take different routes home from work! Go for a jog and explore.

And use your body – learning with the body is really what the brain is designed for as we've seen and so this is an incredibly important way to keep challenging yourself and to keep learning.

Choose activities that will teach your brain useful 'skills' as well. If you want to get more from your brain, then why not learn other languages so that you have more ways to process information? Why not teach yourself to become better at math? Or learn programming?

Because here's the irony – things like this will actually prove to be much more useful in the real world than having a slightly better memory anyway!

The Power of Computer Games

What might surprise you is just how effective computer games can be in all this when it comes to improving your brain power.

Once upon a time, we thought that computer games were bad for children – that they would melt their brains and make them violent (or something). The reality however couldn't be more different.

Computer games have now been shown in studies to improve decision making under stress. Playing action shooters enables us to make better decisions in less time than people who don't play computer games. At the same time, they actually improve visual acuity – they make us more efficient at spotting differences in color and at noticing things on the horizon (which of course is a result of looking out for targets). Computer games can even improve your odds of 'lucid dreaming' – a type of dreaming where you know you're asleep and gain the ability to control your movements and the contents of the dream!

But that's not where the real strength of computer games lies. Rather, computer games offer a very novel kind of brain training because each game is different. Each game uses different controls, which teaches us different motor skills. And each game introduces us to new 3D environments. Sometimes even the physics will change!

Each time you pick up a new game, you're forced to learn the new controls and the new rules. You have to start finding your way around a new environment and you have to change the way you think. This all takes plasticity as new neural networks are made in your motor cortex, as well as in your prefrontal cortex.

Each time you learn a new game, it's like learning a new skill. And you have the exact same releases of dopamine (more so in fact) when you get it right!

In fact, the truth is even more impressive than that. Computer games are addictive because of the release of dopamine. Why is dopamine released when we play games? Because we're *learning*. The brain *loves* learning and if you can make that fun, then suddenly you'll start becoming better at everything!

Smart Drugs Nootropics – But Do They Work?

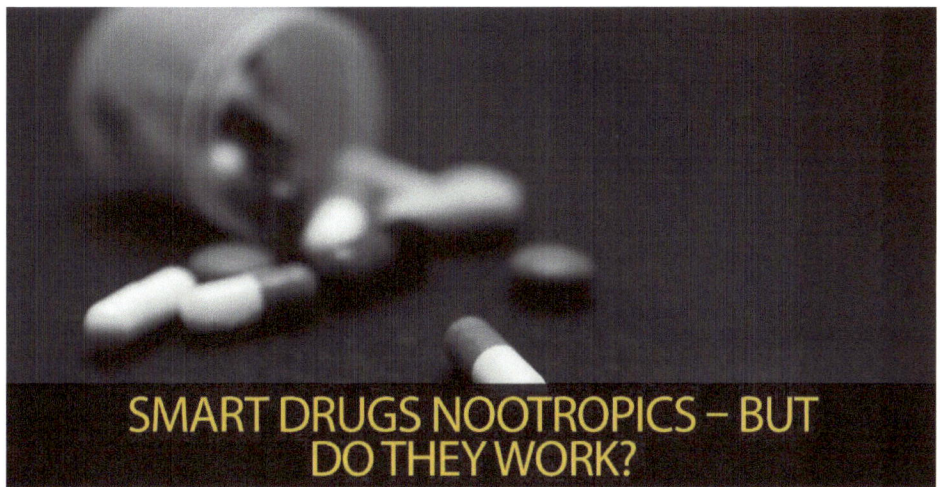

The last chapter has shown us that the best way to strengthen the brain really, is just to *use* the brain and to use it in lots of novel scenarios and to practice things to get better at them.

What a surprise! Strengthening the brain requires effort and practice – just like strengthening the body!

Nothing worth having comes easy, so they say...

But this is going to seem like bad news for a lot of people (even though I basically just told you to play computer games in order to get smarter). Unfortunately, a lot of us don't want to train our brains to get smarter – we just want easy answers. This is the same reason that 90% of people never end up sticking to their training regimes! It's too hard – they want the body, the strength and the confidence but they don't want to put in the work!

Normally, I would say 'too bad'. But as it happens, there *may* be a way you can 'jump ahead' and get the results you want more quickly. And that answer is to use 'smart drugs'. Let's take a closer look at this concept, how it works and whether it is for you.

What is a Nootropic?

A nootropic, also called a 'smart drug', is any form of medication or supplementation that can make you objectively smarter in some capacity. This might mean that you improve your memory, your focus, your creativity or something else. Either way, nootropics are to the brain what supplements and steroids are to the body.

But are they safe? And do they work?

That all depends on what kind of nootropic you intend on using!

Right now, reports tell us that somewhere around 90% of executives and CEOs across America are using nootropics of various descriptions in order to get an edge on their competition. These help them stay up later, be more confident during presentations and generally perform their very best.

One of the most popular forms of nootropic to this end is modafinil. Modafinil is a nootropic that works by increasing the amount of a neurotransmitter called 'orexin' in the brain. This neurotransmitter is at least partly responsible for regulating the brain's sleep and wake cycle, along with various other bodily functions (like appetite and bowel movements). Modafinil was originally designed as a way to treat narcolepsy – a condition that causes people to fall asleep for no reason and without warning – but it was found that it could also improve various other functions like memory, attention and reflexes. This is because it can also increase dopamine, along with various other important neurotransmitters. There are no known side effects and the pill has a half-life of ten hours. So in theory, a CEO can pop one in the morning and then be more alert, more focussed and less sleepy for a whole 10-hour day.

Another example is Piracetam. Piracetam is nootropic that increases acetylcholine in the brain. Acetylcholine is a generic excitatory neurotransmitter in the brain, meaning it generally increases the firing rates of neurons. This results in the brain becoming more alive and subjectively this might make you feel more awake, more alert and more vividly aware of your senses.

Piracetam takes longer to take effect and needs to build up in your system over time – but a lot of people find the effects very pleasant without any notable downsides.

On the other end of the spectrum, you have things like 5-HTP. 5-HTP is 5 hydroxy tryptophan, which is a precursor to tryptophan, which is *itself* a precursor to serotonin. Precursor means 'building block' by the way – meaning that the brain uses these chemicals to make other chemicals.

Serotonin is the feel-good neurotransmitter and is also somewhat inhibitory. All this means that serotonin can help to make you feel relaxed and happy at the same time and thereby combat stress. Serotonin also converts into melatonin (the sleep neurotransmitter), which makes 5-HTP a useful sleep-aid when used just before bed. A CEO might use something like 5-HTP to 'come down' after a stressful day then, to perform better during a presentation by calming nerves, or just to sleep more deeply leading to a more productive day the next day.

Should You Use These Kinds of Nootropics?

So now the big question: should you use these kinds of nootropics?

Of course this is up to you but as general advice, the answer would have to be no. There are no known side effects for something like modafinil or Piracetam but that is not to say that there are *definitely* zero issues. These substances have not been tested for the long term, so no one knows what would happen were you to use them over a 10 year period. Not only that but it's also a little concerning that we don't know precisely *how* many of these nootropics work. 5-HTP we understand – but it's not known precisely *how* modafinil impacts on orexin, only that it *does*. It's completely uncertain how modafinil achieves its *other* benefits meanwhile.

And while there are no 'official' side effects, I can personally tell you that this isn't entirely the case. For starters, it's well known that modafinil will make you need to go to the toilet a lot, while also suppressing your appetite. This is of course a result of it altering the regulation of various bodily rhythms.

I also found that modafinil made me bite the insides of my lips a lot, as well as grind my teeth – likely simply a result of having lots of stimulatory neurotransmitters running around my brain.

Piracetam will give you a headache unless you stack it with choline and many people find that even then, they can end up with both headaches and 'brain fog'. Some people have reported feeling permanent brain fog as a result of using Piracetam.

Modafinil also makes me *so focussed* that it isn't always a good thing. When I use it, I become 'glued' to whatever it is I'm doing. If that's work… great! I will then be completely transfixed on work until I finish. But if I have a quick go on a computer game before I start working, then there's a good chance I'm not going to be able to stop – I'm going to *complete* that computer game before I get any work done!

Likewise, crossing the road can become dangerous as I find myself so engaged in what I'm thinking that I can't properly pay attention to the road or to noises/movement in my environment.

I also find it harder to be creative and this follows seeing as an increase in dopamine and norepinephrine is actually associated with a *decrease* in creativity. We are at our most creative when we are relaxed because this allows our mind to 'wander'. The neuroscience behind this is that our brain is forming new connections between disparate neurons that would normally never be associated – which is how invention happens. But when you're highly focussed, you become too fixated on one thing and this stymies creativity.

The point of all this?

The brain operates the way it does for a purpose. Optimum brain function is *not* about being able to focus on one thing for a long time. Optimum brain function is about being able to switch from one brain state to another *as necessary*. You need to be highly focussed while you're working and then *relaxed* when you're not. You need to let your mind wander when you're trying to come up with new ideas and then focus up when you're asked a difficult question.

When you artificially increase too much of a certain neurotransmitter, you make it very hard to do this and you get 'stuck' in one state. It *feels* optimum but in fact it's just an artificial 'high'.

Another problem with these types of neurotransmitters is that they can actually be addictive because of something called 'tolerance and dependence'. What happens here is that the brain *adapts* to that increased or decreased neurochemical. For example, if you have artificially increased the amount of dopamine in your brain on a regular occurrence, then your brain might respond by *removing* dopamine receptors to make the brain less responsive to it. Alternatively, it might reduce the amount of dopamine you naturally produce.

In short, you now need a bigger dose of the same substance in order to get the same feeling as before. And eventually, your 'baseline' can become so low that you feel bad until you get it! While modafinil and Piracetam aren't officially supposed to be addictive, 5-HTP actually can be and is better avoided for this reason. That and essentially making your brain sleepy is not the solution to heightened social skills and confidence! (No surprise there, really!)

Neurotransmitters Do Not Exist in a Vacuum

As though all that wasn't enough reason, it's also important to recognize that neurotransmitters do not exist in a vacuum. That is to say that any one neurotransmitter you alter, will automatically impact on many others and have other effects on the body. We've already seen for instance that serotonin converts to melatonin and that orexin affects our hunger and bowel movements. Then there's the fact that serotonin links to appetite and that cortisol (also linked with dopamine) affects our testosterone levels.

There are undoubtedly countless neurotransmitters that we have yet to even discover. And what this means is that when you take a nootropic that effects *one* neurotransmitter, you're really make all kinds of untold changes in your brain without really knowing what the consequences of that action might be. For this reason, it's highly advisable to focus on other ways to get your mental upgrade!

What About Caffeine?

But there is a nootropic that most of us *already* use on a regular basis. That nootropic is of course caffeine, which is the secret ingredient in tea and coffee that makes us wake up in the morning and feel more alert. This is just like any other nootropic, the only difference being that it has been around longer and is therefore a little more 'commonplace'.

So how does caffeine works? Basically, caffeine is able to mimic a neurotransmitter in the brain called Adenosine. Adenosine is a by-product of the 'energy process' in the brain. When your mitochondria utilize glucose for energy, they do this by converting it first to ATP (adenosine triphosphate) and then breaking that ATP apart into its constituent parts... including adenosine!

Adenosine builds up throughout the day then as we use our brain cells for thinking, moving and powering our bodies. But this substance is inhibitory and over time makes us become tireder and sleepier. Eventually we become so sluggish that we're forced to go to bed and a good night's sleep is then able to flush our brain of the excess adenosine ready for morning.

What caffeine does is to block the adenosine receptors. Because caffeine is a similar shape to adenosine, it can plug the holes where adenosine is supposed to go and that then prevents adenosine from working its magic. This makes us feel more awake and alert and causes a spike in brain activity. This spike in brain activity then results in a flood of other excitatory neurotransmitters being released, which include dopamine, norepinephrine and more.

So is it safe to use? Will caffeine give you a healthy kick?

Yes and no. On the one hand, caffeine has actually been shown in studies to reduce your chances of developing Alzheimer's and in that sense it is neuroprotective. It does enhance wakefulness and memory and it's relatively very safe. At the same time though, caffeine is *also* essentially 'stress in a cup'. It works by increasing many of our stress hormones and this can decrease creativity (as we've seen), while also causing numerous other problems.

More worryingly, caffeine *is* addictive owing to the mechanisms we described earlier. If you become dependent on caffeine, you'll find you can get raging headaches whenever you go long periods without it.

What's more, it has actually been suggested that what many of us think of as 'morning grogginess', is actually just a withdrawal symptom from caffeine! In other words, we wake up and feel sluggish because we've gone for so long *without* caffeine!

It's really up to you if you take it or not but this is an excellent demonstration of the risks associated with nootropics versus the benefits.

My advice is to think of all these nootropics like laser tools. Stay away from them 90% of the time but when you absolutely *need* to get a huge amount of work done, consider using one just for that day.

Nutrition and Supplementation for More Brain Power

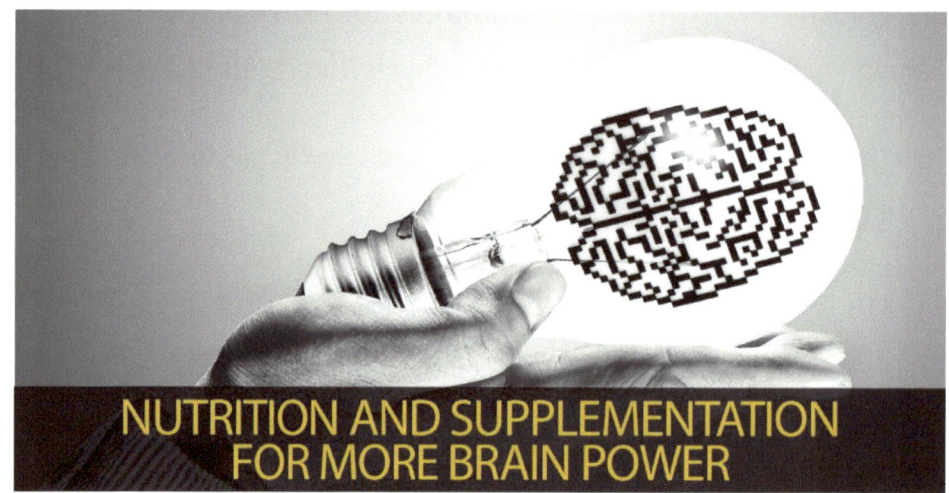

So overall, the cons might just outweigh the pros when it comes to using nootropic to increase or decrease quantities of specific neurotransmitters.

But that is not to say there's no way you can effectively increase your brain power with a little outside assistance. The key is simply to switch your focus to your *long term* brain health rather than trying to get an immediate boost to your intelligence.

And doing this is very easy with the right diet. Diet is absolutely *essential* for brain health and many of us don't realize just how critical it is in this regard.

Let's take a look at just some of the nutrients and supplements that you can use to enhance your brain power...

Amino Acids

Amino acids are the building blocks of protein. When you eat any meat, your brain will break it down into the amino acids and then recombine these to build tissues around your body. These tissues include use in the brain and so consuming more amino acids can be used to actually improve the body's ability to repair and grow the brain!

But this is not where the importance of amino acids ends. Amino acids are *also* crucial for creating many neurotransmitters. For example, l-tyrosine is used to create dopamine, whereas tryptophan (discussed earlier) is used to create serotonin. Others, like l-theanine, can have direct effects on the brain and in this case it's a somewhat calming effect. L-carnitine meanwhile has an energy boosting effect on the brain by increasing the performance of the mitochondria (more on this in a second!).

As we've seen with 5-HTP, it is possible to consume many of these amino acids on their own, in order to trigger immediate changes in the levels of neurotransmitters. However, this leads to imbalances as we've discovered and despite popular opinion, this is never a positive thing.

So instead, the best advice is to focus on trying to get a healthy mix of as many amino acids as possible. By simply eating lots of protein, or supplementing with amino acid products, it's possible to provide the brain with all the materials it needs to create all of the different neurotransmitters as and when it needs them. This then makes it better at entering *every* mental state and ensures that you can maximize your focus, concentration, memory and relaxation all at the same time.

The best way to conveniently get lots of amino acids? To consume plenty of eggs. Eggs are one of the only 'complete proteins' meaning that they contain all of the amino acids that the brain doesn't create on its own. On top of this, they also contain choline, which is the precursor to excitatory neurotransmitter acetylcholine. They're a great source of healthy saturated fat too and seeing as the brain is predominantly made from fat, this is also a very important and beneficial factor.

Vitamins and Minerals

The same goes for countless vitamins and minerals. These too are used to create a lot of the neurotransmitters that are so highly sought after by people trying to enhance their productivity and focus.

Vitamin B6 in particular is used to create a huge number of neurotransmitters. Vitamin C meanwhile is key for increasing serotonin and boosting the mood, while also providing protection against illness (which brings with it cytokines – an inhibitory neurotransmitter).

And there are plenty of other roles for vitamins and minerals too. Iron and vitamin B12 both help with blood flow by producing more red blood cells. Vitamin D helps with the regulation of hormones, especially testosterone. Zinc plays a key role in enhancing neuroplasticity. Magnesium meanwhile helps to combat depression and anxiety.

In short, if you are not getting the micronutrients you need, then you are not giving your brain everything it needs to function optimally.

And this is why you need to *avoid* processed foods. Anything that is very artificial like a Mars Bar, bag of crisps or McDonald's burger will contain calories to fill you up but won't contain the nutrients you need to function. You'll stay alive but you'll feel tired, sluggish and far less productive as a result.

Eat healthy salads, smoothies and lots of fruit and veg and you'll find that you start feeling healthier and alert. The next best thing is a multivitamin and if you get the right one of these then it can do a lot to improve the function of your brain as well as your overall health and wellbeing.

Vasodilators

If you're looking for an immediate brain boost that you can get from safe supplements and foods, then look for vasodilators. A vasodilator is any substance that dilates the blood vessels (veins and arteries). These will allow more blood and more oxygen to get around the body, which in turn will result in more making it to your brain.

A particular favorite among nootropic-fans is vinpocetine because this vasodilator focusses on the brain specifically – and the prefrontal cortex even *more* specifically. This means you're getting more energy right to the part of the brain that you use for planning and problem solving and some people describe the feeling as being like 'a cold shower for your brain'.

Cognitive Metabolic Enhancers

This is a fancy term for anything that increases your brain's energy levels and often this means things that will increase the efficiency of your mitochondria. Mitochondria are the energy factories of your cells. They float around inside the cytoplasm and they use glucose and ATP to power your bodily functions – including brain function!

Numerous things can help your mitochondria to perform better and these include CoQ10, lutein, l-carnitine, PQQ and more. In other words, a mixture of amino acids, vitamins, minerals and all kinds of lesser known nutrients available in supplement form.

Again, the best strategy is just to eat a very balanced and nutritious diet but you can also increase your energy levels further by using creatine.

Creatine is a supplement that is very often used by athletes and bodybuilders. Its main function is to convert used ATP (adenosine and ADP) back into more *useable* ATP. In other words, it recycles adenosine which thereby provides you with extra energy to use in your training.

The more recent surprise though is that this *also* enhances brain function by improving the energy efficiency of brain cells. Basically, it allows the brain to recycle its ATP too, which means you get just a second or two of extra energy at maximum exertion. Studies show that individuals who take creatine get a slight boost to their IQ, so this is definitely a very effective nootropic – and one with zero side effects or risks!

Creatine is produced naturally in the liver and can also be obtains from your diet (sources such as beef). However, the best way to see a significant boost is to use it in supplement form – look for creatine monohydrate.

Omega 3 Fatty Acid

Omega 3 fatty acid is a great antioxidant that is found in tuna and other oily fish, as well as some nuts and various other sources. What makes omega 3 useful for the brain though, is the fact that it can improve 'cell membrane permeability'. Essentially, this means that it makes the cell walls of the neurons just a little more permeable, thereby allowing things to pass through a little more easily. That includes neurotransmitters, nutrients and more – so it essentially makes brain cells more responsive and thereby gives you a slight boost yet again.

Antioxidants

Antioxidants are key for looking after your brain's *long term* health. These include vitamin C, omega 3, resveratrol and tons of other micronutrients.

Essentially, antioxidants work by destroying 'free radicals' – substances that damage cells when they come into contact with them and which can even lead to cancer if they make it through the nucleus and cause damage to the DNA!

Consuming antioxidants is thus a very important strategy for your overall health and will also help you to reduce your likelihood of illness by strengthening your immune system. However, what we're interested in right now is how this can boost your brain power in the long term by protecting brain cells from damage and potentially lowering your chances of developing tumors later in life.

Strategies for Enhancing Brain Elasticity

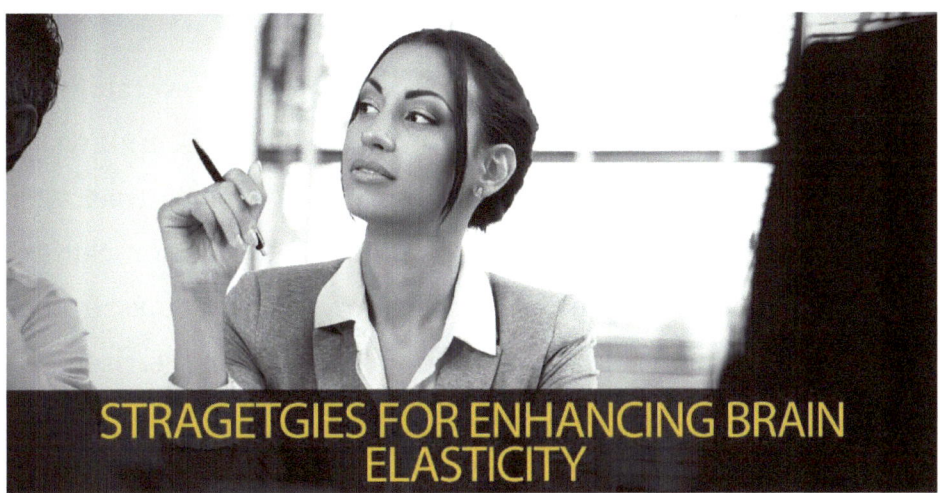

But what about plasticity? Can that be enhanced?

We've already seen a few methods that can help to boost plasticity. The first and most important is to *use* your brain and to subject it regularly to novel stimuli. Likewise, we've seen that dopamine and magnesium are good for plasticity.

But what about nootropics that directly affect this in a big way?

There are a couple of options out there as it happens...

Noots for Plasticity

The first nootropic that can boost plasticity is 'Lion's Mane'. This is a nootropic that acts directly on BDNF to increase the likelihood of new connections being formulated (and which increases when we're presented with novel stimuli).

Lion's mane is actually a mushroom and can be enjoyed as a coffee. Again, there's not a huge amount of information available regarding the mechanisms of action or the long term effects but many people swear by this ingredient as a way to get a mental edge and some unparalleled cognitive boosts.

Another option is to try CILTeP. This is a stack consisting of several different natural nootropic substances including forskolin, artichoke extract, l-carnitine and vitamin B6.The main stars of the show here are the forskolin and artichoke extract, which together increase 'cAMP' in the cells and thereby encourage gene transcription. Suffice to say that it's supposed to improve long-term-potentiation (myelination) specifically and some people find it effective without side effects (including author Tim Ferriss).

tDCS

And then there's 'tDCS'. This stands for 'transcranial direct current stimulation' and basically means that you are running a small current through your brain via conductive pads that are attached to your scalp.

The idea of tDCS is not to cause your brain cells to fire, as there is not enough electricity being delivered to the brain for that. Instead, it is simply to potentiate them, to increase the amount of BDNF and to encourage plasticity. This has been demonstrated to be effective in countless studies and there are again no proven side effects. Pads are placed in different arrangements around the head which are known as 'montages' and these are designed to ensure that specific brain areas get the majority of the current. This then changes the effect of the tDCS – some montages make people more alert and focussed while others can boost the mood or improve sleep. What's particularly interesting is that the effects seem to last about 30 minutes following use.

Just as with stronger nootropics though, it's important to exercise a little common sense here and to realize that there's no such thing as a 'biological free lunch'. Apart from anything else, it's very hard to know precisely the area of the brain that you're stimulating just by looking at a drawing of the scalp! And if you can increase learning in one area of the brain, you could theoretically accidentally cause learning in other parts of the brain too that would be less desirable. Proceed with extreme caution then!

But with all that said, this is definitely an interesting option and especially when you consider a) that there is a huge amount of evidence suggesting that this is a safe way to get a considerable brain boost and b) that there are many commercial products now available that use this technology – and upcoming. The 'foc.us' headset for instance is a product that is designed to boost performance in computer games that can already be purchased online!

Lifestyle and Rhythms of the Brain

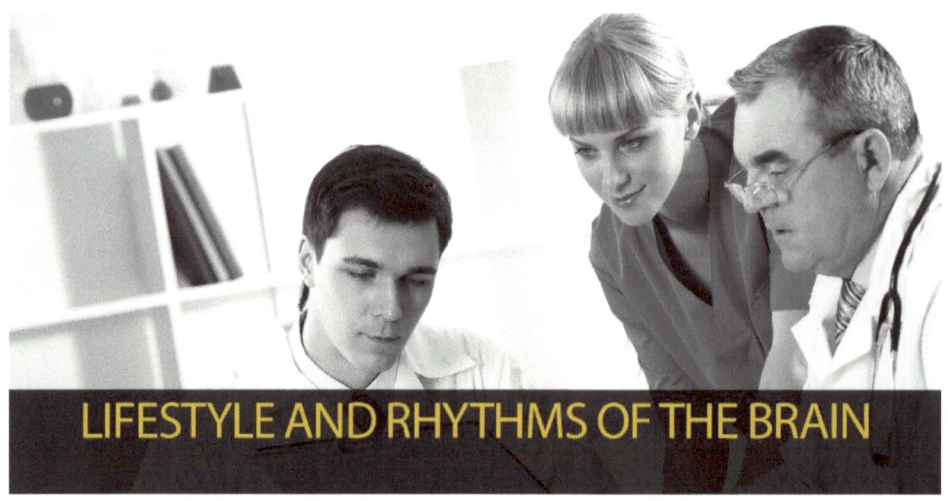

The right nutrition can make a huge difference to your brain power then and so too can dabbling in nootropics and even tDCS as long as you're careful with it.

Then there's the importance of using 'natural' brain training by stimulating yourself with lots of new experiences and challenges.

But despite all this, there is still one alternative method that is *far* more effective when it comes to giving you an immediate boost in your cognitive function, productivity and pretty much every aspect of your brain power.

And that is to *sleep more.*

If you are not getting the best night's sleep possible, then you are not performing at your best and it's that simple. This is because you're still going to have a build up of adenosine in your brain slowing you down and because your brain actually strengthens connections formed throughout the day during the night.

It's also while you sleep that you replenish many of your neurotransmitters and in short, this is an absolutely crucial process for putting you back on top of your mental game. Skip it and you can expect to feel sluggish, slow, forgetful and quite possibly even depressed.

Most people overlook this absolutely crucial factor though and will continue to abuse their sleep – trying to work longer hours or wake up earlier. In the long run, this will be guaranteed to damage your productivity and your brain power... so *get to sleep*.

Tips for Sleeping Better

If you want to improve your sleep and thereby wake up refreshed and better able to focus on what you're doing, then follow these tips...

Have a Hot Bath

Having a hot bath right before bed is a fantastic way to encourage sleep. This will help to relax your muscles which makes it a lot easier to sleep. Furthermore though, it will also help you to produce more sleep-related hormones and neurotransmitters and even to better regulate your temperature throughout the night which also improves your ability to nap.

Have a Regular Sleep Time

Another important tip is to go to bed at the same time every night. Our bodies *love* routine because they are based largely on rhythms. Our sleep rhythm is called the 'circadian rhythm' and is based not only on what time we wake up/go to bed but also on external cues such as the sun and the weather.

If you go to bed at the same time every day, your body will start to find its natural rhythm so that it's ready to sleep when you are and not before.

Use a Daylight Lamp

You can also help this process by giving yourself a 'daylight lamp'. This is a light that is designed to mimic natural sunlight by producing light with a very similar wavelength.

What's more, is that a daylight lamp can be set to come on gradually in the morning to mimic the rising sun. Rather than being rudely 'startled' awake, you'll instead be gradually nudged away by light – as you would have been during your evolution!

Create the Best Environment

This is also why it's so important to have thick curtains. If light comes in from outside, it can reach your brain via the thinner parts of your skull and trigger the release of cortisol to wake you up. But if you keep those curtains opaque then you'll only have the light *you set* to tell your body when to wake up.

Other important tips are to create a quite space to sleep in and to make sure that your bed is as comfortable as possible.

Have a Cool Down Period

Also important is to have a 'cool down' period. This is a period of time during which you're going to avoid anything that might stimulate you. That means you're avoiding all forms of stress but also anything that just wakes you up. So no phones, no computer games and no bright lights. The best way to do this is to read something under a dim light. Reading focusses your inner monologue and thereby prevents your mind from wandering to stressful things. Meanwhile, concentrating on the text will make your eyes heavy which also makes it easier to drift off (and harder not to!).

Routines and Rhythms for Your Brain

The reason this cool down period is so important is because it puts you in a relaxed state ready for bed. This means that you'll have more inhibitory neurotransmitters and fewer excitatory ones.

And this is an important concept to understand because ultimately, both your brain *and* your body are only ever in one of two states: excited or inhibited. You are always either catabolic or anabolic.

Throughout the day, we switch from being ready for bed and sleepy and alert and ready to go. When it gets dark and we're tired at the end of the day, we have cues from the darkness, from the adenosine build-up in our brain and even from dinner (which causes a release of sugar and serotonin/melatonin in the brain). Together, all this slows our heartrate and breathing, reduces brain activity and puts us in a creative and chilled mental state.

In the morning though, bright light causes a flood of cortisol and nitric oxide in the brain which 'boots us up'. Heading to work causes an influx of noise and bright lights to find their way into our brain and stimulate even more adrenaline/norepinephrine to wake us up further. Then comes the coffee for some more cortisol and dopamine and the work for tons of each.

And it's by switching between these two states that the brain is generally able to always perform the right job for the task at hand.

The problem is that we're always sending the wrong signals or trying to force ourselves to stay in one state too long. That's what happens when we play loud video games right before bed, or when we try and force ourselves to work hard at 4pm after we've just eaten.

A big part of performing our best is to understand the importance of letting our brain go through its natural rhythms and trying to work *with it* to get the most from it.

And also important is to try and avoid excess stress. Because when you get *too* stressed – whether that is caused by physiological or psychological factors – this actually causes us to become so wired and focussed that our prefrontal cortex entirely shuts down. This is a state called 'temporo-hypofrontality'. While this can be a good thing sometimes during sports, it's actually the last thing you want during a conversation or when you're trying to be creative!

CBT teaches us a lot of techniques we can use in order to overcome stress and put ourselves into the correct mental state for the job. These include visualizations techniques as well as challenging thoughts that might not be particularly effective.

Meditation is also an incredibly useful tool to this end that you can use to address stress and put yourself in a much calmer and more relaxed state of mind as and when you need to.

The Critical Importance of Exercise

And finally, it is absolutely *essential* that you get lots of exercise if you want to get the most out of your brain. Remember, your brain evolved to help you adapt and survive in the environment via your physical interactions with it. The vast majority of your brain is dedicated to moving your body, so if you want to encourage plasticity then there are few things than learning a new dance or martial art.

What's more though, is that exercise boosts your memory according to studies and stimulates the production of countless crucial neurotransmitters and hormones. Even beyond this, exercise is important to improve your circulation so that you might get more oxygen to your brain.

Final Thoughts

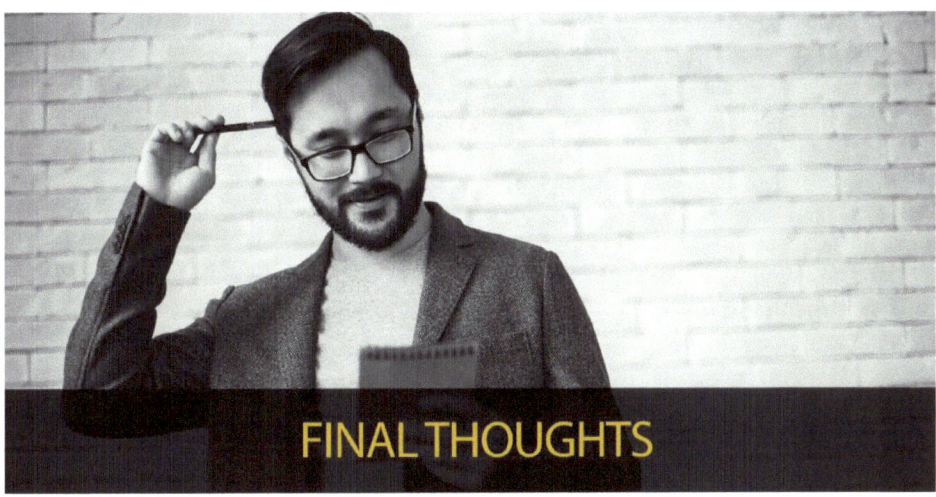

Congratulations on making it to the end! We covered a *lot* of complicated topics there and really did dive in deep with regards to the workings of the brain and how to get the most from it. But if you have made it to this point, then great news is that you now have a much better idea of how the brain works than about 99% of the population.

And hopefully you can also now see the best ways to improve your brain power through training, through diet and through your lifestyle.

Get a nutritious diet, exercise, expose yourself to novel things, learn new mental skills that you can use for thinking, play video games, get more sleep and occasionally consider using nootropics when you really need a boost.

If you do all this and keep mindful of your rhythms and what's going on inside your brain at any given time, then you will be able to tap into the kind of brain power you never knew you had...

About the Author

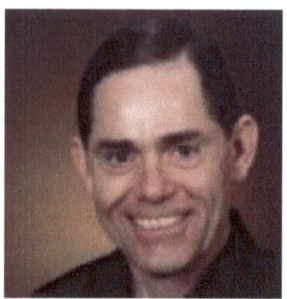

I have published numerous books on Amazon (both for Kindle and in paperback), along with other publishing platforms.

While most of my books are on health and fitness in general, I also write on baby boomer and older citizen health issues and have a recent interest in creating and printing journals/ planners and other printable products. A complete list of our published products on Amazon can be found at https://www.amazon.com/Ron-Kness/e/B0072M6PYO.

Besides my own writing, I also ghostwrite ebooks, books, reports, articles, blogs and do Kindle conversions for clients on a variety of topics. Contact me at Ron Kness Writing for a quote.

Today my wife and I are retired from our careers and live in San Tan Valley, AZ. I now write as a retirement business where you'll find me happily sitting in my office typing away on my laptop as I work on my next book or ghostwriting project . . . that is if we are not traveling on a cruise ship - our new-found mode of travel.